I0477679

Contents

Preface

If you're a migraine sufferer or simply interested in migraines, then this will be a crucially significant book for you.

This book covers information about types of migraines, a brief history of past approaches to migraines, current day treatments, the biology and mortality of migraines and natural medicine approaches. It also opens a window into Siddha - a 10,000-year-old medical system used in Southern India that offers a lifestyle change and in doing so can cure migraines as well as many other more serious medical issues.

Imagine being able to live your life with less migraine attacks. What if you could have more days in a month where you feel well, you're not in pain with a throbbing head, you don't have as many visual disturbances, you don't have to call in sick to work, you don't lose days of your life just lying in bed; because you feel well, healthy, able to think clearly, and you're migraine free? Finally, imagine being able to treat and prevent your migraines in a natural way, which do not have the unpleasant side-effects experienced with all the chemicals.

In this book you'll learn about:

- Conventional pharmaceutical treatments, but some of the negative side-effects these can have.
- The biology and mortality of migraines
- Natural treatments and preventatives for migraines

You'll learn the hidden truth behind 2 different herbs you can take for migraines. You'll discover 2 essential oils that can ease migraines.

You'll find a little-known way to combat migraines using Siddha and this one approach may well change your life.

Introduction

Migraines affect 10 -15% of all adults in the population[1]. They can be tremendously debilitating, depending on the type of migraine and this can cause a very severe throbbing headache which can be on one or both sides of the head, sickness, sensitivity to light and noise, visual disturbances, they can affect speech (making it become slurred) and can even make the body have a weakness. People may experience a migraine for 4 – 72 hours. If people have a migraine for 14 days or less per month, this is episodic migraine. If it's experienced for 15 days or more out of a month, this is chronic migraine.

Different Types of Migraine

There are many different types of migraine that people can suffer from. The most common form is a migraine that does not have an aura; 70-90% of people that experience a migraine do so without an aura. Others may have a migraine with an aura and this means that they may have various visual disturbances where they see coloured spots or sparkles, flashing lights, or blind spots in their vision. If people have a migraine for more than 15 days in a month, this is known as a chronic migraine. Some ladies may have migraines that are in sync with their menstrual cycle. If temporary weakness is involved on one side of the body, this is a hemiplegic migraine. Some migraines may have a brainstem aura, this was previously called a basilar-type migraine. There may be a connection between migraines and vertigo. Some children may have abdominal migraines. There may be a connection between cyclical vomiting syndrome (CVS) as a child and then suffering from migraine attacks when older[2].

Approaches to Dealing with Migraines

---

[1] Song Guo. Breakthroughs in Migraine Treatment.
http://blogs.biomedcentral.com/on-medicine/2018/03/09/breakthroughs-migraine-treatment/
[2] 'Types of Migraine' – The Migraine Trust.
https://www.migrainetrust.org/about-migraine/types-of-migraine/

Once migraines have been diagnosed, there tends to be 4 key aims:

1. To reduce how often migraines occur
2. To reduce how severe the migraine is
3. To reduce the length of the migraine
4. To ensure that the patient has the best quality of life they can

Simple Lifestyle Changes to help Prevent Migraines

Simple things such as ensuring you eat a balanced diet and eating regularly can help. Ensuring you get enough regular sleep can also be useful. Incorporating exercise can help you to suffer from less migraines. Drinking enough water throughout the day is always going to be beneficial to your health. There are certain known foods and drinks which can sometimes trigger migraines, so avoiding these will be sensible. Some known triggers include dark chocolate; citrus fruits such as oranges and lemons; caffeine; artificial sweeteners (especially those with aspartame in them); alcohol, especially red wine and beer, alcohol is also dehydrating; Monosodium glutamate (MSG); cured meats which release nitric oxide into the blood; aged cheeses containing tyramine; pickled or fermented foods, which also contain tyramine; ice-food/drinks that can cause 'brain-freeze' stabbing pains; salty food because of the sodium in them.[3]

---

[3] '10 Foods That Trigger Migraines' – HealthLine - https://www.healthline.com/health/foods-that-trigger-migraines#caffeine

Chapter 1: A Brief History of Medical Discoveries

In a 1986 journal article in the Journal of Neurology, Neurosurgery and Psychiatry, JMS Pearce traces the history of the Migraine from Hippocrates and 3,000BC[4] where the migraine is described as "a sever pain in one half of the head associated with disturbance of sight." The medical descriptions of migraines carry on through Celsus (A.D.30); Arataeus (A.D.81); Galen (AD 131-201) ….

Trepanning

In the past if people had headaches, then a hole would be put in the skull to relieve pressure on the brain. This was something that cavemen did in the 8th Century BC, and it became popular again in the 1600s, with people having their skulls drilled.[5] Other people have suggested that skulls were opened throughout people's lives to 'release evil spirits.'[6]

1960s – Serotonin and Triptans

Jumping forward quite a lot in time, in the 1960s it was found that people who had migraines, often had quite low levels of serotonin,

---

[4] JMS Pearce. Historical Aspects of Migraine. Journal of Neurology, Neurosurgery and Psychiatry. 1986.
https://jnnp.bmj.com/content/jnnp/49/10/1097.full.pdf
[5] Chris Stokel-Walker, 5 Bizarre and Scary Historical Headache Curres,
http://mentalfloss.com/article/52689/5-bizarre-and-scary-historical-headache-cures (2013).
[6] Katherine Foxhall, 'Migraine Myth: Drilling Holes in the Skull was Never a Cure – But it was Long Thought to be.' (2018)
https://www.independent.co.uk/life-style/health-and-families/migraine-cure-trepanning-trepanation-drill-holes-skull-ancient-humans-stone-age-a8243381.html

which prevents pain and helps to constrict blood vessels.[7] As a result of this, drugs called Triptans were discovered (see the next chapter for more information on these).

1990s – Cortical Spreading Depression and Transcranial Magnetic Stimulators

People who suffered migraines were found to have a hypersensitive occipital cortex, making these people more sensitive to light, noise and other triggers. When something triggers it, it is known as cortical spreading depression, which causes vessels to dilate and for prostaglandins and other substances to be released.[8] A transcranial magnetic stimulator which sends an electric current through a metal coil can be held against a person's head, so a magnetic pulse creates an electric current in the nerves of the head. Patients reported that this did cure their migraines that they experienced at the time, and after a few treatments their migraines stopped because the brain has 'forgotten' the pattern of electrical activity that causes the migraine.

---

[7] Marshall Jon Fisher. The Biology of …Migraines. Discover.
http://discovermagazine.com/2004/aug/biology-of-migraines
[8] Marshall Jon Fisher. The Biology of …Migraines. Discover.
http://discovermagazine.com/2004/aug/biology-of-migraines

Chapter 2: Current Day Treatments for Migraine Headaches

If you've been diagnosed with migraines, there are 2 types of medicines you could be prescribed:

1. **Pain-Relievers** – to stop the symptoms of the migraine during the attack. Taken when you have a migraine.
2. **Preventative Medicine** – designed to stop or at least reduce the frequency that you get migraines, you would take these usually on a daily basis.

Pain-Relief

If the migraine is mild, this could include drugs such as Aspirin, Ibuprofen, Advil, Motrin IB and Paracetamol. Acetaminophen and Tylenol may also help. There's a prescription pain reliever in suppository form called Indomethacin. Sometimes these drugs are combined with caffeine and marketed for migraines. If the migraine is severe however, these are not likely to be effective.

Triptans

Triptans are a medication used for treating migraines, they work by making the blood vessels constrict and blocking the pain pathways (see Chapter 4 on the Biology of Migraines, for more information on this). You can get Triptans in tablet form, nasal sprays, and injections. Some well known Triptan medications include: Zolmitriptan (Zomig); frovatriptan (Frova), sumatriptan (Imitrex), rizatriptan (Maxalt), naratriptan (Amerge) almotriptan (Axert) and eletriptan (Relpax).[9] A

---

[9] Migraine. May Clinic. https://www.mayoclinic.org/diseases-conditions/migraine-headache/diagnosis-treatment/drc-20360207

single table that contains both sumatriptan and naproxen sodium (Treximet) can be more effective to relieve migraines than just taking one of these.

Ergots

These drugs combine Ergotamine with caffeine, they tend to be used if people have a migraine for more than 2 days. Ergotamine however does come with the side effects, that it may make the person more nauseas and cause vomiting, which is never nice at any time, but when your head is already pounding, this exacerbates the situation. There is an ergot derivative which has less side effects, called Dihydroergotamine (D.H.E 45, Migranal). This can be in the form of a nasal spray or injection.

Preventative Medicine

People that experience more than 4 migraine episodes per month often consider preventative medicine and more so if their migraines last longer than 12 hours; if pain relief doesn't help and if your migraines include auras, numbness or weakness.

Some preventative medicines include: Beta blockers, Antidepressants, Anti-seizure drugs; Botox and Aimovig. Beta blockers are a cardiovascular drug, they can take a number of weeks to fully get into your system to a point where they make a difference. There are also calcium channel blockers that can be useful in migraines with auras. Even if you don't have depression, some Tricylcic antidepressants may reduce migraines by changing serotonin levels, a common tricyclic to be prescribed is amitriptyline, but this drug can cause side-effects of tiredness, a dry mouth, weight-gain and constipation amongst others. Anti-seizure drugs can reduce the frequency of migraines, but again, these come with a whole host of possible side-effects, from dizziness, weight gain, nausea, hair-loss, issues with memory and concentration, diarrhoea etc. Botox may be useful, administered by a doctor into the forehead and neck muscles, but this needs to be done every 3 months. Aimovig (Erenumab-aooe), is a drug which you self-inject once per month, and this can inhibit a molecule which causes migraines. See the next section on this.[10]

Erenumab

In 2017 a drug called Erenumab was presented as managing to 'half' the amount of migraines that people experienced.[11] It was a phase III clinical trial. Erenumab is a monoclonal antibody that blocks the CGRP receptor. In the trial there was a placebo assigned to half the patients too. Erenumab was administered to half the trial patients via a subcutaneous injection. The higher the milligram dose the more effective the reduction of migraines. Patients who took the drug had much more of a decrease in migraines, in comparison to the placebo group. But, within the placebo group, still 26.6% of those experienced a 50% or greater reduction in their migraine days. The trial was carried out on almost 1,000 patients. It could make a significant difference to people around the world. In the UK, more than 8.5 million people experience migraines each year, which is a higher number than those people affected by epilepsy, diabetes and asthma combined. Due to sick-days taken because of migraines, this can cost the UK economy more than £2bn per year![12]

---

[10] Migraine. Mayo Clinic. https://www.mayoclinic.org/diseases-conditions/migraine-headache/diagnosis-treatment/drc-20360207
[11] Honor Whiteman. Migraine breakthrough: new drug halves attacks. https://www.medicalnewstoday.com/articles/320224.php
[12] Migraine drug could halve the length of attacks, study shows. https://www.theguardian.com/science/2017/nov/30/migraine-drug-erenumab-could-halve-the-length-of-attacks-study-shows

Anti PAC receptor mAbs

In March of 2018 Dr. Song Guo in Copenhagen wrote in the *Journal of Headache and Pain* about a small molecule which is related to migraines. It is called a Pituitary Adenylate Cyclase Activating Peptide (PACAP). It can be discovered in the central nervous system.[13] If the calcitonin gene-related peptide (CGRP) is treated this can be effective in treating migraines.

There have been phase II and III trials, where CGRP function-blocking monoclonal antibodies (mAbs) which are antibodies that are made up of replica immune cells and this has shown to be a good preventative measure for both episodic and chronic migraine. Dr. Song Guo believes that the anti-PAC receptor mAbs are more effective than anti-CRGP mAbs because the PAC1 target is more specific to migraines.[14]

---

[13] Song Guo. Breakthroughs in Migraine Treatment.
http://blogs.biomedcentral.com/on-medicine/2018/03/09/breakthroughs-migraine-treatment/ [accessed 22nd Sept. 2018].
[14] Song Guo. Breakthroughs in Migraine Treatment
http://blogs.biomedcentral.com/on-medicine/2018/03/09/breakthroughs-migraine-treatment/

Chapter 3: Statistics on the Success of Treatments

- The drug 'Erenumab' is reported to halve the length of migraine attacks.[15]
- Topomax an epilepsy drug from Ortho-Mcneil Pharmaceutical, has half of all patients reporting a 50% reduction in frequency of migraines, and more than a quarter have reported a 75% reduction.[16]
- According to the Migraine Trust, "less than 50% of migraine patients are satisfied with their current treatment. The majority self-medicate using non-prescription (over-the-counter) medication and do not seek medical help."[17]
- Migraine/chronic headache was found to be the second most frequently identified cause of short term absence (47%) for non-manual employees.[18]
- The World Health Organization class severe migraine attacks as among the most disabling illnesses, compared to psychosis, dementia and quadriplegia. [19]

---

[15] Migraine drug could halve the length of attacks, study shows. https://www.theguardian.com/science/2017/nov/30/migraine-drug-erenumab-could-halve-the-length-of-attacks-study-shows and Whiteman, Honor. Migraine breakthrough: new drug halves attacks. https://www.medicalnewstoday.com/articles/320224.php

[16] Marshall Jon Fisher. The Biology of ...Migraines. Discover. http://discovermagazine.com/2004/aug/biology-of-migraines

[17] Facts and Figures. The Migraine Trust. https://www.migrainetrust.org/about-migraine/migraine-what-is-it/facts-figures/

[18] CBI, Pfizer. Healthy Returns? Absence and Workplace Health Survey 2011.

[19] World Health Organization. Atlas of headache disorders and resources in the world 2011.

Natural Treatments

- In a study of 31 patients who took 150mg of CoQ10, 61% reported at least a 50% reduction in the days they had a migraine, with no side-effects reported either.
- In a study with 42 patients, migraine sufferers took CoQ10 three times a day, 100mg compared to a placebo group. The CoQ10 was shown to be three times more effective than the placebo.

Chapter 4: The Biology of Migraines

Migraines seem to be related to the constriction then sudden dilation of blood vessels in the brain. According to Johns Hopkins these changes in blood flow don't 'initiate the pain but may contribute to it.' [20] It's thought today that hormones such as serotonin and estrogen can also play a part in sensitivity to pain.

It has been found that a calcitonin gene-related peptide (CGRP) and a pituitary adenylate cyclase-activating polypeptide (PACAP) can be responsible for dilating blood vessels in the brain and causing a migraine attack. There is a peptide called PACAP38 which is a key molecule, a vasodilator, responsible for migraines and cluster headaches.[21] PACAP38 activates the PAC receptor.

This can be why, often, Triptans are a form of medication used in migraine relief, because Triptans do the opposite, they constrict the blood vessels and block pain pathways.

It is also believed that some brain cells can trigger chemicals such as serotonin and these too narrow blood vessels. In some people with a sensitivity when serotonin or estrogen levels change in the body, this can cause a migraine. Serotonin affects men and women, but estrogen levels only affect women, and this can be why women get migraines associated with monthly changes in estrogen.

There are certain things that can trigger migraines:

- Tiredness and changes to sleep patterns
- Bright glaring or flickering lights
- Changes to the weather

---

[20] How a Migraine Happens – Johns Hopkins Medicine - https://www.hopkinsmedicine.org/healthlibrary/conditions/nervous_system_disorders/how_a_migraine_happens_85,P00787
[21] Song Guo. Breakthroughs in migraine treatment. http://blogs.biomedcentral.com/on-medicine/2018/03/09/breakthroughs-migraine-treatment/

- Certain foods/drinks – caffeine, dark chocolate, oranges, cheese etc.
- Stress and other emotions
- Exposure to light or smells
- Biological hormonal shifts

Whereas in the past migraines may have been considered a blood vessel disorder, they're now beginning to be considered a sensory perceptual disorder.[22] Two-thirds of people with acute migraine attacks have 'allodynia' which makes people sensitive to certain stimuli.

In 2013 the Wellcome Trust Sanger Institute, made a media release, which said that researchers identified some of the biological roots of migraine from a large-scale genome study. There were 12 genetic regions associated with migraine susceptibility. 8 of these were connected to brain circuits. 2 were connected to areas responsible for maintaining healthy brain tissue.[23]

---

[22] Emily Underwood. The Science of Migraines.
https://www.sciencemag.org/news/2015/02/science-migraines
[23] Getting to Grips with Migraine. Media Release. Wellcome Trust Sanger Institute.
http://www.headachegenetics.org/sites/default/files/Getting%20to%20Ogrips%20with%20migraine.pdf

Chapter 5: Migraines and Mortality

From the evidence, it seems to be that migraine sufferers who also have auras with their migraines, are at the greatest risk of mortality from cardiovascular, or coronary heart-disease or haemorrhagic stroke. If people have co-morbidities with migraines, such as depression, alcohol-related illness, or mental disorders this can increase their risk of mortality.

Some migraines may cause lesions in brain tissue, called 'infarctions' – this would be a complication of migraines. If people smoke or take oral contraception, this may also increase the risk.[24]

Auras and Cardiovascular or Coronary Heart Disease

A 2011 study by Markus Schurks et al, looked at 'Migraine and Mortality: A Systematic Review and Meta-Analysis' and what they found was that if people suffer from migraines with auras, this increased the chances of mortality from Cardiovascular or Coronary Heart Disease. [25] This was similar to a study the previous year by Larus S Gudmundsson et al, 'Migraine with aura and risk of cardiovascular and all cause mortality in men and women: prospective cohort study'[26] The purpose of their study was to determine whether having migraines in mid-life was associated with cardiovascular disease and similarly it was determined that people

---

[24] Emily Underwood. The Science of Migraines.
https://www.sciencemag.org/news/2015/02/science-migraines
[25] Markus Schurks. Migraine and Mortality: A Systematic Review and Meta-Analysis.
https://www.ncbi.nlm.nih.gov/pmc/articles/PMC3175288/
[26] Larus S. Gudmundsson et al. Migraine with aura and risk of cardiovascular and all cause mortality in men and women: prospective cohort study. https://www.bmj.com/content/341/bmj.c3966

who had migraines with auras were at risk of mortality from cardiovascular disease compared to people with no headaches.

Auras and Haemorrhagic Stroke

Studies have looked at cardiovascular causes of mortality linked to migraines and into migraines with auras being linked to a higher risk of mortality for haemorrhagic stroke. People who have migraines with auras had "more than twice the risk for haemorrhagic stroke compared with women with no history of migraine."[27]

Women and Migraines, plus Statins

In 2016 the Telegraph's science editor Sarah Knapton reported that "women with migraines have a higher risk of dying from heart problems and statins could help lower the chances of an early death,"[28] however, statins as a drug can come with a whole host of their own awful side-effects, of causing nerve damage and pain in people's legs, making it difficult to walk. The statistic showed that women with migraines were "50 per cent more likely to die," from cardiovascular disease. [29]

---

[27]Mark Borigini, M. D, Migraine Headache and Increased Mortality. Psychology Today. (2011)
https://www.psychologytoday.com/gb/blog/overcoming-pain/201102/migraine-headache-and-increased-mortality
[28] Sarah Knapton. Migraines raise risk of heart attack and early death, scientists find. The Telegraph.
https://www.telegraph.co.uk/science/2016/05/31/migraines-raise-risk-of-heart-attack-and-early-death-scientists/
[29] Mark Borigini M.D. Migraine Headache and Increased Mortality. Psychology Today.
https://www.psychologytoday.com/gb/blog/overcoming-pain/201102/migraine-headache-and-increased-mortality

Comorbidities with Migraines – Alcohol Related Illness

In a very current study from July 2018, Tomor Harnod et al, looked at the 'Survival outcome and mortality rate in patients with migraine: a population-based cohort study.' The study was carried out in Taiwan, but it would be interesting to see if it applied to other populations. For people who had migraines they had comorbidities with alcohol-related illness, depression and mental disorders which were highlighted as risk factors for subsequent mortality and in particular, the alcohol-related illness as a comorbid factor "significantly increased the mortality risk."[30]

---

[30] Tomor Harnod. Survival outcome and mortality rate in patients with migraine: a population-based cohort study. (2018)
https://thejournalofheadacheandpain.biomedcentral.com/articles/10.1186/s10194-018-0889-4

Chapter 6: Migraines and Natural Medicine

Many people wish to try a more 'natural' preventative medicine, or treatment for their migraines. There are various vitamins, supplements and herbs which have been found to be useful.

Vitamins and Supplement

Amongst the recommended vitamins and supplements to help with migraines are: Vitamin D, Coenzyme Q10, Magnesium and Riboflavin.[31]

Vitamin D

It has been studied whether people who are deficient in Vitamin D, may be more prone to suffering from Migraines.[32] The study showed that high levels of serum 25-OH-D3 resulted in a greater number of migraines (this was a positive weak relationship) but no significant relationship was shown between Vitamin D and migraine severity.

Coenzyme Q10 (CoQ10)

Coenzyme Q10 is something that the body naturally makes within its cells, it helps to give cells energy. It is also an antioxidant which can reduce damage to cells. You can also buy Coenzyme Q10 as a supplement and some studies have shown it may be beneficial to reduce or prevent migraines. There are certain foods that are rich in CoQ10 too, such as roasted peanuts, pistachios, sesame seeds, mackerel, rainbow trout, soybean oil, broccoli, boiled egg,

---

[31] 'Supplements and herbs- The Migraine Trust - https://www.migrainetrust.org/living-with-migraine/treatments/supplements-and-herbs/
[32] Tayebeh Mottaghi et al. The relationship between serum levels of vitamin D and migraine. https://www.ncbi.nlm.nih.gov/pmc/articles/PMC3743325/

strawberries, canola oil, beef, chicken, and cauliflower. If you take it as a supplement that you could buy from a health food shop and it is best to take it with food.

There have been two studies which have investigated CoQ10 and migraines – the first study was quite small, with just 31 patients. They took 150mg of CoQ10 and 61% reported at least a 50% reduction in the days they had a migraine, with no side-effects reported either.

In another study again fairly small, with 42 patients, migraine sufferers took CoQ10 three times a day, 100mg and were compared with a placebo group. The CoQ10 was shown to be three times more effective than the placebo. But, there were some side effects of stomach upset and a skin rash.[33]

Magnesium

It has been shown that people who suffer from migraines can be quite low in magnesium. One study showed that if people regularly took magnesium this could reduce migraines by 41.6%. Another study showed that taking daily magnesium supplements could prevent menstrual related migraines.[34]

Riboflavin

In a 2004 study, high doses of riboflavin were found to be effective in preventing migraines. The study took place at a specialist outpatient clinic, where patients took 400mg of riboflavin and the migraine frequency reduced from 4 days a month, to 2 days a month. [35]

---

[33] Coenzyme Q10 for migraine. https://migraine.com/migraine-treatment/natural-remedies/coenzyme-q10/
[34] Magnesium and Migraines - https://www.healthline.com/health/magnesium-for-migraines#magnesium-and-migraines
[35] Boehnke C – High-dose riboflavin treatment is efficacious in migraine

Herbs

Feverfew

In 2004, research was carried out and in 3 out of 5 trials Feverfew was found to be effective in treating migraines.[36] In the remaining 2 trials, there was no difference between Feverfew and the placebo. Feverfew is taken as a prophylactic to prevent migraines. People have said that after taking Feverfew, they've had fewer migraine attacks. Some people have said that they haven't had any at all.

Feverfew can come in freeze dried capsules, of around 250mg. It is possible for you to grow your own feverfew and have some of the leaves in salad or sandwiches, but it can have a bitter taste. You can dry them yourself too then seal them in an airtight container.

Butterbur

Butterbur contains Petasin and Isopetasin, which reduce inflammation and are considered to reduce inflammation and prevent or reduce migraines.[37] Butterbur can be bought as capsules, tinctures, powders and teas.

However, the Neurology Times in 2015 published an online article by two Doctors who expressed some safety concerns at the use of butterbur as a migraine preventative.[38] Clinical trials have taken place

---

prophylaxis: an open study in a tertiary care centre. (2004)
https://www.ncbi.nlm.nih.gov/pubmed/15257686
[36] 'Feverfew' – The Migraine Trust.
https://www.migrainetrust.org/living-with-migraine/treatments/feverfew/
[37] Butterbur. https://migraine.com/migraine-treatment/natural-remedies/butterbur/
[38] Thomas P. Bravo, MD and Bert B Vargas, MD. Migraine Preventative

and it did indeed seem to reduce the occurrences of migraines by almost half, with the only adverse side-effect being 'burping'. It was also shown to be more effective than a placebo in migraine prevention. But, the safety concern comes from the fact that butterbur contains pyrrolizidine alkaloids (Pas) which causes hepatoxicity in humans and can be mutagenic and carcinogenic in animal studies. So, the suggestion is that if this is used, then the Pas need to be removed from it.

Essential Oils

Peppermint

If you have peppermint as an essential oil, you'll need to dilute it with a carrier oil such as 'coconut oil' and then you can apply some to your temples, which can help to relieve the pain of a migraine.[39] Other ways that the oil could be used are a few drops added to a bath, or a bowl of steaming hot water in the room, so that the vapours fill the air. It could be added to a massage oil. It could also be placed into a diffuser.[40]

Lavender

Lavender as an essential oil can be used for migraine relief. Lavender is very soothing and calming, it is thought that it acts as a sedative. A

Butterbur Has Safety Concerns. http://www.neurologytimes.com/headache-and-migraine/migraine-preventative-butterbur-has-safety-concerns (2015)
[39] Peppermint Oil - https://www.healthline.com/health/essential-oils-for-headaches#-peppermintoil
[40] Peppermint Oil for Migraine and Headache Relief - https://www.healthline.com/health/migraine/peppermint-oil-for-migraines#how-to-use

study in *European Neurology* shows how inhaling lavender essential oil could be an effective and safe way to treat migraine pain. In another *Journal of Herbal Medicine* migraine sufferers who used lavender for three months, said that the frequency and severity of their migraines had reduced.[41] To inhale lavender oil, you could add 2 - 4 drops of oil to a bowl of boiling water and inhale the vapours. Or you could add some oil with a carrier oil and massage it into the skin.

Acupressure

Acupressure is classed as a complimentary and alternative treatment to pharmaceuticals to treat migraines. It stems from traditional Chinese medicine and the belief that by applying pressure to parts of the body, pain will be relieved. Acupressure is along the same lines as acupuncture, only acupuncture uses needles, and this doesn't. In Chinese medicine chi is the life force that flows through the body in certain pathways. When pressure is applied at certain points on these pathways (also known as meridians) it's thought the body can be balanced and disease and pain alleviated. Pressure is usually applied with fingers. There are specific acupressure practitioners, or this is something you can do yourself. Practitioners of acupressure believe that it works and relieves migraine symptoms.
Some other medical practitioners think acupressure may work because it improves circulation, relieves stress and tension and may increase the release of endorphins. Regardless of the reason though, if it works this has to be good news for migraine sufferers.

There are a number of acupressure points that have been effective in relieving migraines. These include: The gallbladder 20 (or Feng Chi); gallbladder 21 (or Jian Jing); Large Intestine 6 (or He Gu); Pericardium 6 (or Nei Guan); and the Triple Energizer 3 (or Zhong Zhu). If you're

---

[41] How to Use Lavender Oil for Migraine Relief.
https://www.healthline.com/health/migraine/lavender-oil-for-migraines#4

pregnant, acupressure may not be advisable, in case it induces premature labor.[42]

Yoga

In 2014 a study was carried out by Ravikiran Kisan et al, looking at the effect of yoga on migraines.[43] The results showed that migraine frequency and intensity was reduced more when people were involved with yoga therapy, the yoga also helped to enhance the vagal tone, decrease the sympathetic drive and create better cardiac autonomic balance. Yoga can help to reduce stress, and stress could be one of the factors that cause migraines. A gentle yoga to start which could be Hatha yoga, which is a lot of breathing exercises to start, then yoga poses, and ends with a resting period. It would be sensible to get a proper yoga teacher, rather than watching a video, because they can encourage you to hold your neck and head correctly, so that this doesn't cause any tension or damage. It is important to drink plenty of water throughout and post classes.[44]

Siddha

Siddha has a long history (more than 10,000 years) and is still in wide use in Southern India. There are Siddha hospitals, clinics and surgeries as well as Ashrams and other more spiritual or holistic

---

[42] Acupressure. https://migraine.com/complimentary-and-alternative-therapies/acupressure/

[43] Ravikiran Kisan et al. Effect of Yoga on Migraine: A comprehensive study using clinical profile and cardiac autonomic functions. International Journal of Yoga. https://www.ncbi.nlm.nih.gov/pmc/articles/PMC4097897/

[44] Yoga for Migraines. https://www.webmd.com/migraines-headaches/yoga-migraines

practitioners that provide a range of services based on lifestyle, diet, exercise, natural medicine and spirituality. This holistic approach is widely accepted as prolonging life considerably with far fewer health or medical complications than you would expect in the mainstream.

"In Siddha, Migraine is being known as Otrai thalaivali, which is characterized by severe head ache at one side of the head, later it spreads to entire head, visual or neuralgic aura, vomiting and prostration. Head ache in certain cases, will be active for several days. Mandai idi, Mandai soolai, Thalai nokkadu, Thalaikkuthu, Kabala soolai are some of other terminologies used for migraine".

"According to modern side, though aetiology is unknown for migraine, genetic predisposition, hormonal influences, dietary precipitants, psychological stress are considered as some of factors which precipitates migraine. In Siddha, Vayu plays a major role and with the support of either Vatham or Kapham, manifests migraine. Improper food habits and personal habits also participate in the onset of disease. Siddha also deals about another two varieties of migraine pointed by the Siddhar "Yugi muni", and they are Soorya vartham and Chandra vartham. Head ache starts from morning and will be persisted till evening in case of Soorya vartham where as in Chandra vartham pain will be felt entire night and disappear in the morning. Pain also will be felt in the areas like eye, in between eye brows, base of the nose in certain cases and neuralgic involvement also seen"[45].

"In Siddha, in addition to internal medicines, much importance is also given for external applications like medicated oil bath, Poochu, Nasyam, Pugai. Kasthuri mathirai, Linga chenduram, Maha elathi gulikai, Gowri chindamani, Ayakantha chenduram, Arumuga chenduram are some of the Classical preparations usually prescribed by Siddha doctors. For external use, Arakku thylam, Chukku thylam, Sirobara nivarana thylam, Chithira moola thylam, Aswagantha bala laksha thylam, Chandanathi thylam, Nochi thylam are being used as bath oil. Nasyam also giving much relief during attack and Chukku thylam, Nochi thylam and Peenisa thylam are used for this purpose. Since this migraine results from the impairment of vatham, in the beginning of treatment gentle purgation will be advisable. But these medicines could be taken only under medical supervision"[45].

People such as "Swarmi G" have created a system within Siddha that has a strict holistic focus. Swarmi Gs' approach is to treat the whole person using a range of methods that include Acupressure, Acupuncture, Yoga, Divine healing, Energy exchanges, 100 herbal oil baths (Siddha) Meditation, Sanskrit sloga and mantras, Verma manipulation, Topical Herbal Medicine (Siddha) Ingested Herbal Medicine (Siddha) Body Rubs with essential herbal oils (Siddha) Massage with 300 Herbs mixed oils, Modification of diet and creation of a diet plan - food as a medicine, Exercise and repetition movements including traditional South Indian dance, Nature exposure such as a waterfall shower and mediation at a hill station, Self-empowerment and education on self-respect and proper maintenance of weight and body structure and Activation of the bodies immunities and teaching how to maintain this.[45]

"Swami G is able to create a vast range of medicines and treatments for all manner of ailments. Of particular interest is his knowledge on how to treat cancers using only natural medicine and in this respect he has successfully treated a wide range of cancers including skin cancer, blood cancer, lung cancer, liver cancer and pancreatic cancer to name a few."[46]

"Natural medicine is a term commonly misunderstood and certainly in the context of Siddha medicine the term 'natural medicine' requires a person not in the knowledge of Siddha to redefine what natural medicine actually is. Whatever occurs naturally in nature (I mean everything) is considered to have a medicinal use either alone or in combination with one or more other natural elements. When you start to fully understand Siddha you will realise that the medicinal cupboard of a Siddha practitioner is so vast it defies comprehension."[47]

---

[45] Swarmi G - http://www.sreenaturallycureyou.com/index.html
[46] Swarmi G - http://www.sreenaturallycureyou.com/index.html
[47] Swarmi G - http://www.sreenaturallycureyou.com/index.html

Ayurveda – as a component of Siddha or as a derivative

According to Ayurveda, migraines may mostly be associated with an aggravated vata dosha caused due to mental stress or insomnia. The dry nature of vata can make you dehydrated, leading to stiffness of muscles and constipation that trigger a headache[48].

Unlike the broad approach of Siddha the medicinal aspects can be seen in isolation or as a component of Siddha. The Ayurveda medicine approach is more than 5,000 years old and is widely practiced within India and around the world.

"Ayurveda is "non-symptomatic medicine", says Peter Gowan from the Australasian Ayurvedic Practitioners Association. He says it aims to instruct people how to live so they don't get sick, rather than waiting for illness to develop.

What is ayurvedic medicine?

Ayurveda is an Indian health practice thought to be more than 5000 years old. It consists of a number of disciplines, including aromatherapy, diet, herbal medicine, acupuncture, yoga, massage, meditation and balancing of energies.

The word "ayurveda" is translated from Sanskrit to mean "the science of life".

Ayurveda proponents believe earth, water, fire, air and space make up the universe. Chyle (a fluid composed of lymph and emulsified fats), blood, flesh, fat, bone, marrow and semen are believed to be the body's primary elements. Many traditional practitioners believe semen is the most precious and should be preserved through celibacy.

---

[48] Home Remedies for Migraine: 6 Superb Ways to Cure the Pain - https://food.ndtv.com/health/home-remedies-for-migraine-6-superb-ways-to-cure-the-pain-1620822

Ayurvedic practitioners use the terms "vata", "pitta" and "kapha" to describe your body type and determine a course of treatment/diet. Vata types are said to be thin and bony with restless minds; pitta have a moderate physique with muscular limbs and an alert mind; and kapha have broad frames, long limbs and are calm and patient."[49]

---

[49] Whimn – my body and soul -
https://www.bodyandsoul.com.au/health/health-news/what-is-ayurvedic-medicine/news-story/8955c25c2d4966f8815e0c8595eca857

Conclusion

Migraine sufferers have been the victim of many dodgy practitioners, drug companies and other practices that have not really helped the sufferers. Migraine suffering is as long as humanity itself and the one word is not helpful in describing the diversity of suffering that is titled as Migraine.

One helpful practice that may assist some people is simply walking bare foot in the morning on dewy grass. Whenever it occurs in the morning go and walk in it. This will earth your body out and remove any excess or confused electrical energy in your body. The reason I know it works is that my mother was told this many years ago by a Naturopath and when she tried it, it significantly changed her life for the better.

Simple things like walking in dewy grass at the start of the day and drinking a different beverage with breakfast may just solve your problem, while for others it may do nothing. This is the troublesome nature of humanity and migraine. And it is why there are so many treatment options and so many disappointed people still suffering and are frustrated at the lack of proper diagnosis and treatments.

From my investigations, I can honestly say that the natural medicine pathway holds the key to the migraine solution. By simply walking in the dewy grass each morning, removing soft drinks and lollies from your diet will change your body age within weeks and lead you to a longer happier life. Similarly, by not smoking cigarettes and not consuming excessive alcohol will further improve your outlook. If you were to walk in dewy grass, remove soft drinks, lollies, smoking and excessive alcohol for 3 months and then see how your migraines go. Record what happens on a calendar. Be strict with yourself and record exactly what happens.

After this, remove coffee form your diet and introduce alkaline water. Alkaline water should be mild – about ph 8.5 to 8.8 and you can get a recipe from the internet or purchase it from the health food store –

natural is better of course. You need to properly hydrate yourself and in this respect 2 litres of normal tap water per day is the target. A normal drinking cup is 250ml. So 8 cups of water per day. Introduce Alkaline water slowly and monitor your bodies reaction to the new item in your diet. Over time try to mix it 50/50. So, half the water you drink is tap water and the other half is alkaline water. Try this for 3 months, record the results and see what happens. If at any time things get worse simply remove the element that you introduced and wait for things to normalise.

You can see from the above 2 paragraphs that fixing your problem does not necessarily cost you any money. In fact, it may save you a small fortune.

Finally, if all else fails, I have one further solution. If you are at wits end and cannot function properly and are over all the medication and all the rubbish you have been fed, send an email to the following email address and I will put you in touch with Swarmy G. Be aware though, this person is not your normal run of the mill doctor. He is a tea total vegetarian and has never smoked or drank alcohol. He is very strict and you will have to travel to India and stay with him in the Ashram. I have done this and I can tell you it will change your life – totally. 2 weeks is enough I think in normal circumstances but of course you may fall in love with the food and the culture and want to stay longer – up to you and of course, how much you can afford.

admin@sreenaturallycureyou.com

You can also see the Ashram etc on the web -
www.sreenaturallycureyou.com

If you decide to go there and you have purchased my book/guide I can arrange a discount for you. The daily rate for migraine, or any serious treatment, costs like a holiday. The things that impressed me were the airport transfers, **the food** (vegetarian even though I am a carnivore) the accommodation, the sightseeing, the blunt honesty, down to earth people and approach, Shiva and the explanations etc. Very good intervention in all. Of course, the main outcome is the cure and you will get that if you do as you are told. Also, the follow up medication or diet plan etc. Life changed, no more pain and eyes opened wide.

Remember this, when you are self-medicating with natural medicine or food as a medicine etc, you need to have discipline and be very strict with yourself. It is your life after all so be careful what you do with it.

If you decide to go to India and meet Swarmy G you need to take notes. It would be an idea to take a tablet or Ipad etc and take screen shots of the plants and medications and make notes of what he tells you. He is not big on handouts. His mind is full of Siddha medications and so forth. When he talks it is not from a book – straight from the head.

Finally, let me know how you go. I need to know good and bad and if there are any issues in this guide or book that should be updated etc.

I hope you get some relief and that this book has helped you.

PS: I am now 61 and basically migraine free. I still get the occasional moving target in my eyes if I have eaten liquorice. But no pain and days off! Damned shame as I love liquorice and days off!

Good Luck!

Glossary of Terms

Migraine prophylaxis - Migraine prevention

Phonophobia – sensitivity to and discomfort from loud noises/sounds

Photophobia – discomfort from light exposure to eyes, physical sensitivity

Placebo – no real effect, 'dummy' pills

Bibliography

'10 Foods that trigger Migraines' – HealthLine.
https://www.healthline.com/health/foods-that-trigger-migraines#caffeine

Acupressure. https://migraine.com/complimentary-and-alternative-therapies/acupressure/

Boehnke C – High-dose riboflavin treatment is efficacious in migraine prophylaxis: an open study in a tertiary care centre. (2004)
https://www.ncbi.nlm.nih.gov/pubmed/15257686

Borigini, Mark, M.D. Migraine Headache and Increased Mortality. Psychology Today.
https://www.psychologytoday.com/gb/blog/overcoming-pain/201102/migraine-headache-and-increased-mortality

Bravo, Thomas P. MD and Bert B Vargas, MD. Migraine Preventative Butterbur Has Safety Concerns.
http://www.neurologytimes.com/headache-and-migraine/migraine-preventative-butterbur-has-safety-concerns (2015)

Butterbur. https://migraine.com/migraine-treatment/natural-remedies/butterbur/

CBI, Pfizer. Healthy Returns? Absence and Workplace Health Survey 2011.
Coenzyme Q10 for migraine. https://migraine.com/migraine-treatment/natural-remedies/coenzyme-q10/

Facts and Figures. The Migraine Trust.
https://www.migrainetrust.org/about-migraine/migraine-what-is-it/facts-figures/

'Feverfew' – The Migraine Trust.
https://www.migrainetrust.org/living-with-migraine/treatments/feverfew/

Fisher, Marshall Jon. The Biology of …Migraines. Discover.
http://discovermagazine.com/2004/aug/biology-of-migraines

Foxhall, Katherine, 'Migraine Myth: Drilling Holes in the Skull was
Never a Cure – But it was Long Thought to be.' (2018)
https://www.independent.co.uk/life-style/health-and-
families/migraine-cure-trepanning-trepanation-drill-holes-skull-
ancient-humans-stone-age-a8243381.html

Getting to Grips with Migraine. Media Release. Wellcome Trust
Sanger Institute.
http://www.headachegenetics.org/sites/default/files/Getting%20to%
20grips%20with%20migraine.pdf

Gudmundsson. Larus S. et al. Migraine with aura and risk of
cardiovascular and all cause mortality in men and women:
prospective cohort study.
https://www.bmj.com/content/341/bmj.c3966

Guo, Song. Breakthroughs in Migraine Treatment
http://blogs.biomedcentral.com/on-
medicine/2018/03/09/breakthroughs-migraine-treatment/

Harnod, Tomor. Survival outcome and mortality rate in patients with
migraine: a population-based cohort study. (2018)
https://thejournalofheadacheandpain.biomedcentral.com/articles/10
.1186/s10194-018-0889-4

How a Migraine Happens – Johns Hopkins Medicine -
https://www.hopkinsmedicine.org/healthlibrary/conditions/nervous_
system_disorders/how_a_migraine_happens_85,P00787

How to Use Lavender Oil for Migraine Relief.
https://www.healthline.com/health/migraine/lavender-oil-for-
migraines#4

Kisan, Ravikiran, et al. Effect of Yoga on Migraine: A comprehensive
study using clinical profile and cardiac autonomic functions.

International Journal of Yoga.
https://www.ncbi.nlm.nih.gov/pmc/articles/PMC4097897/

Knapton, Sarah. Migraines raise risk of heart attack and early death, scientists find. The Telegraph.
https://www.telegraph.co.uk/science/2016/05/31/migraines-raise-risk-of-heart-attack-and-early-death-scientists/

Magnesium and Migraines -
https://www.healthline.com/health/magnesium-for-migraines#magnesium-and-migraines

Migraine. May Clinic. https://www.mayoclinic.org/diseases-conditions/migraine-headache/diagnosis-treatment/drc-20360207

Migraine drug could halve the length of attacks, study shows.
https://www.theguardian.com/science/2017/nov/30/migraine-drug-erenumab-could-halve-the-length-of-attacks-study-shows

Mottaghi, Tayebeh, et al. The relationship between serum levels of vitamin D and migraine.
https://www.ncbi.nlm.nih.gov/pmc/articles/PMC3743325/

Peppermint Oil - https://www.healthline.com/health/essential-oils-for-headaches#-peppermintoil

Peppermint Oil for Migraine and Headache Relief -
https://www.healthline.com/health/migraine/peppermint-oil-for-migraines#how-to-use

Swarmi G - http://www.sreenaturallycureyou.com/index.html

Schurks, Markus. Migraine and Mortality: A Systematic Review and Meta-Analysis.
https://www.ncbi.nlm.nih.gov/pmc/articles/PMC3175288/

Stokel-Walker, Chris. 5 Bizarre and Scary Historical Headache Cures,
http://mentalfloss.com/article/52689/5-bizarre-and-scary-historical-headache-cures (2013).

'Types of Migraine' – The Migraine Trust.
https://www.migrainetrust.org/about-migraine/types-of-migraine/

Underwood, Emily. The Science of Migraines.
https://www.sciencemag.org/news/2015/02/science-migraines

Whiteman, Honor. Migraine breakthrough: new drug halves attacks.
https://www.medicalnewstoday.com/articles/320224.php

World Health Organization. Atlas of headache disorders and resources in the world 2011.

Yoga for Migraines. https://www.webmd.com/migraines-headaches/yoga-migraines

www.ingramcontent.com/pod-product-compliance
Lightning Source LLC
Chambersburg PA
CBHW070930220526
45468CB00005B/1726